This book is made out to all Endometriosis sufferers around the world and to everyone who helped me over the years.

I was an early bloomer, while the average girl gets her first period at age twelve the mass majority will get their periods anywhere from ages eight through to fifteen. I got my first period at age seven. from ages seven to nine, I had irregular bleeding, but once I turned nine, it became regular and has been that way ever since.

My mum knew something was wrong straight away because of how much pain I was in; I spent the first seven years of having my period missing school, being in and out of the doctors in pain only to be told I was putting the pain on, being asked if I was trying to get out of school because I was getting severely bullied, once they even wondered if there were problems at home.

When I was ten, I was put on my first birth control pill because my periods were lasting anywhere from ten to fourteen days of nonstop bleeding. While I would love to put what birth control I have been on, I sadly can't; I have been on all birth control pill options in New Zealand, both funded and non funded in the duration of six years.

When I turned fourteen, I finally found a doctor who would listen to me, my grandmother also suffers from Endometriosis, and my symptoms were a lot like hers. This doctor listened to everything I had to say and sent a referral to a gynecologist. Keep in mind that I live in New Zealand, right at the bottom of the south island, where not much in the way of medical staff is located. The mass majority of Endometriosis specialists are in the north island.

At my first appointment, my grandmother came along with me, and this gynecologist was actually from Christchurch, so this was a one-off appointment. She listened and was very pushy, kept trying to get me to have a Mirena placed. I wasn't feeling really confident in that appointment, but to my surprise, there was a list of Endometriosis symptoms up on the waiting room wall, and I had all but one of those symptoms, which was painful sex, but at this point, I hadn't even had sex so I didn't know if I would have that symptom or not.

My next appointment was with the guy I would see for the rest of the time; he was a lot more understanding and even sent a form to my doctor for ultrasounds; he gave me a new form for birth control which I had to try for three months, this was my third birth control. I also got a refill on my painkillers as well as a new painkiller. I was now on paracetamol, Tramadol and ponstan.

I eventually got my ultrasound which showed my left ovary had a chocolate (ovarian endometriomas) cyst. From there, we started trying more and more birth controls. My pain started to get worse after my fourteenth birthday, and after getting pregnant at fourteen and losing my babies in a miscarriage, the pain becomes consistent every day and flaring up way more around ovulation and my period.

By fifteen, I was put into southern health school because I was missing more than two weeks of school a month due to the pain putting me behind on all my school work. Southern health school is a school for kids who can not attend regular school because of illnesses. My mental health was shot, I had multiple suicide attempts though some were from trauma, not just my Endometriosis; I had an overnight stay with a twenty-four-hour suicide watch and was later put into Pact (a programme to help people recovering from mental illness) for two weeks.

My gynaecologist didn't want to do surgery on me due to my age which was also putting a damper on my health. Having to live every day in pain is not easy. While my pain was ever changing by the hour, the best way I can describe it is on lower pain days, it feels like a dull stabbing pain all over my back and abdomen. On higher pain days, it feels like sharp stabbing pains with a burning hot knife that is twisting inside me while the rest of my body is covered in barbed wire that is getting pulled tighter and tighter. Another way I have described the pain is as if an alien is inside my body and ribbing itself out of my abdomen, pulling all my organs out as it comes.

By sixteen, I was put onto a new pain medication called Amitriptyline at a dosage of 25mg. I was instructed to take one tablet daily for two weeks and then increase it to two tablets a day thereafter instead of all the other medications I was on. I was no longer on birth control because I had gone through all the pills he could offer me. I refused and still to this day refuse to get any implants in or the Mirena, I know they work wonders for some women, but it is just not for me; I considered the depo shot, but after being on the pill form and not being able to stop bleeding I decided that wasn't the right option.

 Something I found extremely interesting one day when ranting about my pain to another lady with Endometriosis was her saying I couldn't be in as much pain as I was because I was refusing implants. It both surprised me and upset me; out of everyone in the world, I thought another lady who was suffering the same thing as I would understand that not every type of birth control works for everyone and it is a choice, I wasn't willing to get anything placed long term after knowing what has happened with all the pills and knowing how sick I got on them. Yes, you can get them out, but it isn't something I wanted to do, knowing the risk of it being the same is so high. It was also upsetting to hear her say I can't be as bad as I say I am all because I choose not to get something fitted. This was my first real encounter with realising that even in our community, some women are horrible. We all have off days and pain but saying something that we hear all too often to another suffer hurt and bad.

I think now is the right time to talk about my reactions to the birth control so you guys can understand where I was coming from. I have only ever been on one birth control that has ever worked for me, and that was my first birth control. I was on that; I want to say a year and a half before it stopped working. They put up my dosage to see if that would work, which it didn't ; after that it was all downhill.

I am not going to go through a list of symptoms for each birth control because we would have a very long book otherwise, but I will do an over hall of symptoms, starting with the ones that happened on most of the birth control and ending with the ones that occurred on only one type.
I got extreme nausea, some even making me vomit and not just in pain but because of the birth control itself.

I had an increase in pain, sometimes it was worse than what it was off the birth control, and sometimes it was just making my bad pain days more often.

Headaches, I am used to headaches, ones that used to make me miss class or gym because of them, but these headaches were weird; they wrapped around my head and would cause a ringing in my ears. Each part of my head hurt at different levels of severity.

Increase in bleeding, some of them made me bleed a lot more than average; I don't want this book to be TMI, but this is a book about Endometriosis, and extreme bleeding is a regular thing for other women and myself. But I would be going through almost twice as many products as I would typically, and that is a lot.

Breakthrough bleeding, I will be touching on something similar then this in a second, but I actually got random bleeding outside of my period on some of the birth control, something that had never happened to me before.

At times my period actually went irregular. Now going from regular periods to going irregular was very scary for me. I didn't know what was going on, and because of the random bleeding, I was ruining a lot of underwear. Typically on my period, I wear black or grey clothing and black underwear. But when it is coming out of nowhere, it was ruining a lot of my clothing, and some of it was my favourite pairs, and they couldn't be saved.

Period not stopping. This one was the depo in pill form; I was on it for an entire month, and while I had a few of the above symptoms, everything was going pretty well until my period came, there was so much blood, and it wouldn't stop, I think I was on day ten of my period when I said fuck it and stopped taking the pills, two days later the bleeding stopped, I tried the following month again to see if it was a one-off thing, but it did it again so I just knew I couldn't take it without my period not stopping.

Touching on the similar thing to the breakthrough bleeding. Both my gyno, doctor and a doctor in accident and emergency advised me to take my pills back to back to skip a period altogether. I tried this for a number of months on different kinds of birth control, and it seriously wouldn't work. The day my period was due, it came even if I wasn't on the sugar pills. I don't know why I couldn't skip my periods, but apparently, my body doesn't like not having a period, so it physically wouldn't allow me to.

In addition to being on loads of birth control, I have also been on loads of pain medications. Panadol, Codeine, Tramadol, Ponstan, Ibuprofen, I did try Amitriptyline, but as the time I am writing this, I didn't give It a fair shot because of all the side effects I got like feeling hungover and not being able to wake up in the morning and having to get up for appointments and to look after animals and get up though night when they need to go to the toilet, it just wasn't going to work. I tried all of these in different dosages and even mixing them in various combinations to try and help.

I personally find it hard to explain to people what Endometriosis is, not only because it is hard to put into words what it is but also because whatever I say, some people want to argue. I usually tell people it is a chronic illness that affects one in ten women that causes extreme pain and other horrible symptoms, but some people think that because they haven't heard about it that it isn't authentic or because I am so young that I don't know what I am talking about. I never claim to know all the answers, nor do I in this book; I am trying to spread awareness on the horrible condition because it has gone on too long of it being called taboo.

Explaining something to people that don't have a chronic illness or not having a period altogether is hard; at least when talking to females, it is easier to explain in a way because you can talk about how many pads you go through a month etc. and they will understand that way guys, on the other hand, are mostly grossed out by that. But even by woman, I have gotten very upset about some of their comments; I am no cry baby, but when you are in pain daily, being told you can't possibly be going through that or that you need to toughen up can hurt a lot. A way that I like to tell people is by a bunch of photos on my phone, explaining what it is, what it affects and what not to say to a sufferer.

Endometriosis has taught me not to take things for granted. It is a huge wake-up call when your health gets in the way of your day to day life so that you can't even do some of the most basic tasks in life; I never knew it would be so difficult to put one foot in front of the other at times. I didn't ask for this, nor do I wish this on my worst enemy; this isn't living, and It never will be, and it is unfortunate to know my health has ruined some of my dreams and goals. If you or someone you know is a sufferer, spread awareness, help them, don't judge anyone with how they cope, feel or act because we never know what someone's reasons are or what lead them to do the things they have done.

The pain I feel with Endometriosis is brutal to explain and is often very TMI. The reason it is hard to explain is because the pain changes in different parts of my cycle and also varies depending on where the pain is and what I have been doing that day. If I was to work out, for example, I might find that my pain is worse than if I had just woken up, but this isn't always the case, and sometimes, after working out, the pain is less than it was a week prior with me just waking up.

Some of the ways I may explain the pain is that it is sharp, it burns, it's a stabbing pain, the pain is radiating all throughout my body. One way I told my mum that she found it pretty funny was that it felt like an alien was inside me, and it was trying to rip itself out of my body. Other ways are that there is barbwire wrapped around my body being pulled tighter and tighter while someone is setting my body on fire and stabbing me repeatedly; that one is the one I typically feel sadly.

Sometimes instead of people asking what the pain feels like, they will ask me what symptoms I get. now, this is a hard one because it depends on the day and month, and some will only come for a few days every six months, but overall the symptoms I have experienced are:
- vomiting and nausea
- tiredness/ insomnia
- pain during sex
- bloating
- anal pain

- cervix pain
- pain when I have a full bladder
- pain before/ during a bowel movement
- back pain when sitting too long
- not being able to walk
- pulling inside when moving
- pain when urinating
- heaving bleeding
- constipation
- periods that range 24 to 32-day cycles
- periods that last between 3 and 15 days.

Obviously, throughout the years, I have gained a lot of these symptoms, and some have gotten worse while others have gotten better. For example, my cycle usually is 26 days and last five days, while over the years, the bleeding has gotten worse, and so have the anal, cervix and pain during sex.

On July 22nd 2020, after ten long and painful years of suffering from Endometriosis, I went in for my surgery and finally got an official diagnosis of Endometriosis. I was never told what stage I have.

I had my surgery really early in the morning. I believe I was the third patient, and I was randomly put through the private hospital around where I live without having to pay a dime because of going through the long waiting list with the public health system. I was taken into the theatre around 10:30 in the morning after not being allowed to eat from midnight. Everything was really calm, and they talked me through everything that was happening; they even let my mum be in the room with me to make sure I was okay until I was ultimately out. My experience with my lap was a lot better than the experience I remember from my first surgery, which was to remove my tonsils and adenoids.

I know right before I went to sleep, I imagined them saying things that were not being said.

It took me a bit longer than usual to wake up. Still, in saying that, I hadn't really gotten much sleep before my surgery because I had a friend at the time stay the night unexpectedly. We were up until four in the morning talking, so I only got two hours of sleep before I was woken up to go to the hospital.

After I got to my recovery room, I felt sick and almost started to throw up on multiple occasions. But after about an hour and a half from when I finally got to my recovery room, I was discharged and allowed to go home.

They were only able to remove one lesion from memory because the rest they couldn't get without damaging some of my organs just because of where it was growing.

When it comes to recovery, it went better than expected. I was put on A five-day course of antibiotics which landed up giving me thrush, but my surgeon was expecting that, so they had also prescribed a one-off pill for thrush to kill it, which worked perfectly.

 During recovery, I did land up throwing up once from pain because I tried to wean myself off painkillers before I was ready to. I couldn't sleep on my side for three weeks without crying in pain, and I spent the first-week sleeping sitting up with pillows all around me because if I laid down, I couldn't get up, and I couldn't lean down for a week and a half either.

I did push myself a lot in my recovery thinking I should be able to do more quicker then I actually could. Sadly my surgery offered me no relief from the pain, not even temporarily.

Endometriosis is a condition in which tissue that usually lines the uterus grows outside the uterus. There is no known cause of the condition, and Endometriosis affects every woman differently. That means that no one treatment will work for everyone.

Most of the time, Endometriosis is found
on the bowels or bladder,
on the tissues that hold the uterus in place,
behind the uterus,
on or under the ovaries,
on the uterus,
Fallopian tubes,

in rare cases, it has been found in other parts of the body, such as
the lungs,
brain,
ribs,
spine,
eyes,
skin,
in the hip and shoulder sockets.

A study was done in Scotland on 13,655 people, 8,280 of these women were healthy, and the other 5,375 women had Endometriosis. When the research team analysed the data from the women, they found that Endometriosis increased the risk of miscarriage by 76%. The data was presented at the annual meeting of the European society of human reproduction and embryology and showed that most pregnancies were fine. Still, there was a higher rate of complications.

The odds of an ectopic pregnancy went from the usual 0.6% to 1.6% in women with Endometriosis, and premature birth was increased by 26%. In comparison, the need for a cesarean section was increased by 40%. It is thought that Endometriosis changes the way the uterus functions, and more inflammation is damaging the pregnancy.

Endometriosis can affect a menstruating woman from well before the time of her first period to well after menopause. The severity of pain a woman feels is not linked to the amount of Endometriosis she has. Some women experience no pain even though their Endometriosis is stage three or four which means that the affected areas are large or there is scarring. On the other hand, some women have severe pain even though they have only a few small areas of Endometriosis like stage one or two.

Some of the symptoms a woman will experience are but are not limited to:
painful or disabling menstrual cramps,
lower back pain,
intestinal and/or pelvic pain,
pain during or after sex,
painful bowel movements or painful urination around or during the menstrual period,
spotting or bleeding between periods,
large blood clots,
heavy bleeding,
infertility,
fatigue,
Bladder troubles like interstitial cystitis,
ain in other places such as the lower back,
Pain at other times, e.g. with ovulation or intermittently throughout the month,
irregular periods.

Pain is not expected when you have your period; discomfort is, but something could be wrong if it causes actual pain.

Something people who do care about the pain some women go through want to know is how they can help. This question does depend on the person and how they suffer, which makes answering this question when asked by anyone hard, and you can only really answer for yourself, not the whole community because everyone is different.

The best way to help someone with Endometriosis is to talk to the sufferer you want to help, ask them how it affects them, but don't pressure them for answers because not all sufferers are ready to talk out about it and ask them how they cope and how you can help them manage. Do your own research, Remember, they will have their down days, and that's okay. The key is to make them feel like they are not alone. If they are in a flare-up and need pain medication, then offer to get it for them and a drink to take it with and understand what they are going through and don't try and push yourself and your help on them.

Regarding what other help there is out there for sufferers, there isn't a lot due to the misinformation and it being taboo.
There are many groups on Facebook that are related to Endometriosis. Still, some of these have ladies that are mean and think they know everything when we only learn so much because there isn't that much information out there.

There is an app with thousands of women suffering, and that is the only place I go consistently because I find they are less judgmental on what you have and haven't tried. Instead of advising without knowing anything about how it affects you, they try to realise you are not alone in this battle.

I think there are in-person support groups you can go to in some places, but not many businesses have them, so the best option would be to search for endometriosis support groups near you.

Many people have come to the misconception that Endometriosis will kill you if untreated, which isn't true. Endometriosis is classed as Benign, meaning it has no risk to your life.

Other people believe it is a disability or not a disability, but it depends on the person. Although Endometriosis is not commonly thought of as a disability, some of the symptoms associated with Endometriosis can severely impact a person's life. Suppose you are no longer able to work or earn a living because of your Endometriosis. In that case, you may be eligible to receive Social Security Disability benefit even here in New Zealand.

I occasionally get asked what treatment options are out there and sadly there are not a lot of options for treating Endometriosis.

None of the options out there will get rid of Endometriosis forever because there is no cure to this illness; It grows back!

The treatments available are only used to manage the symptoms, slow down the growth of endometriosis and remove the lessons for temporary relief.

The options out there include:

Medications (birth control, pain killers, pills to put you into early menopause etc.)
Laparoscopic surgery
At-home treatments to manage pain (heat, bed rest, diet etc.)

It isn't easy to live with Endometriosis with the consistent pain and overwhelming symptoms, but it isn't cheap either. You can get health insurance, but for many women in New Zealand and Australia, we find that trying to get health insurance after being diagnosed or even having suspected Endometriosis on your medical profile makes things extremely hard.

The annual healthcare cost burden in the USA associated with Endometriosis was estimated to be $22 billion in 2002, of which $17.3 billion was due to direct medical costs (outpatient and hospitalisation) and $4.7 billion was due to indirect costs (loss of productivity). Endometriosis costs the UK economy £8.2bn a year in treatments.

The average direct cost per patient with Endometriosis:
1 year post-diagnosis: $1730.72,
Two years post-diagnosis: $758.09.
Cost per surgical procedure: Ranging from $14,564.73 (vaginal hysterectomy) to $26,002 (other peritoneal adhesiolysis).
Laparoscopy: $21,268.26
early menopause pills: $845 per month
birth control: $0.00- $50 per three months
pain medication: $2.00-$60 per prescription

This is all variable from country to country and state to state.

So as you can tell, there is a very high cost associated with Endometriosis which could contribute to the added stress and mental health issues that women experience I myself included.

Every kid, at one point or another, will be asked, 'what do you want to be when you grow up?' My answer was almost always the same for years at a time.
"I want to be a teacher," I would say, then it turned to
"I want to be a lawyer," then
"I want to be a midwife" these things would last years; I would research the university or school I wanted to go to, and I would try and learn as much as possible about the career so that I would be as prepared as possible, but as I got older. The pain worsened. I gave up on my dreams, but one stuck when I was a toddler, and I refused to give it up, being an author and mother.

As the Endometriosis got worse, I focused more and more of my attention on my writing. It isn't easy, but I still hold onto it. Many sufferers try and hold onto as many of their dreams as possible, but they too know it isn't always easy, and sometimes they have to let go and focus on something else.

Especially when bosses always struggle to understand, we can't help but occasionally take sick days off because of the pain at times. I have heard of women losing their jobs because of it, which isn't right; we don't choose to be in so much pain as not to be able to move or to throw up uncontrollably from the pain.

I started to try and set myself up for the future. I started at ten years old after suffering from the pain that no one could tell me the cause of for four years.

I started writing, started a YouTube channel, and researched how to work from home and survive. I tried many failed attempts at doing surveys for money, tried to get paid sponsorships and more to be able to make a liveable income.

I never imagined growing up that even my dream of being a mother would be affected by Endometriosis.

During pregnancy, I never got relief, I was always sore and sick, and after my daughter was born, my Endometriosis flared up badly; my pain became uncontrollable. I was put back onto Cerazette, which also landed up with me getting put on Fluoxetine because the birth control made me depressed but just like before, the birth control didn't help. Because of breastfeeding, I couldn't take any of my regular pain meds, not that they would have helped anyway, so I just suffered day in and day out in unbearable pain trying to raise and look after my child.

When she was five months old, I landed up in a month-long flair-up with five days of being unable to move because of the pain. It made me feel worthless. The one thing I always wanted was to be a mother, and while I got that dream after losing twins when I was younger, it was more complicated than I ever could have expected with Endometriosis. I considered dying and leaving her with her father to escape the pain.

Sadly this is all too common, which is something I wish I had known, the amount of misinformation about pregnancy and Endometriosis made me believe that things would be better even temporarily after she was born, but I was wrong; I'm just lucky my doctor listened enough to get me onto antidepressants to help with my emotions, and I had a sound support system which is something a lot of women don't have the luxury of having.

I am now thankfully able to function with my daughter, but that isn't always the case for a lot of women. A lot has been taken away from me because of my endometriosis, but I no longer allow my endometriosis to define me.

I took my writing more seriously, started an online store, became regular again with YouTube and started a podcast about writing while also finding ways to manage parenting with endometriosis so I can be the best person I can be. Yes, when her father and I split, I was on the benefit to survive, but I'm not ashamed of that because it allowed me to work on what I needed to.

Some women aren't as lucky, though. Many lose their jobs because of Endometriosis and have to push through pain until they give up and their mental health gets the best of them.

Talking about mental health that leads me to the next topic I want to talk about.

Every woman is different when it comes to mental health and endometriosis. Still, a study was done on a bunch of women who were asked to complete a questionnaire in their own words that assessed the effect of endometriosis on education, work and social well-being, and endometriosis-associated symptoms and health-related quality of life.

The study showed that endometriosis affects work in 51% of women, and 50% of women stated that it impacted relationships. Despite care management, 59% of women continued to have painful periods, 56% of women had painful intercourse, and 60% had chronic pelvic pain. Endometriosis decreased the quality of life in all eight dimensions of the SF-36v2 (an instrument to measure health-related quality of life) than norm-based scores derived from a general US population.
Painful sex, chronic pain, and the number of co-morbidities had an independent negative effect on both the physical and mental components of quality of life.
Other factors that correlated with these women's quality of life were affected work (negative) and having a partner present for support (positive).

Experts in the field are actively investigating the association between endometriosis and the development of mental health conditions like anxiety and depression. Several studies have shown that endometriosis, and its related symptoms and experiences, can lead to impaired mental health and a decreased quality of life.

The association is more robust in women who don't have an understanding partner to support system and those who experience severe symptoms.

However, any woman with endometriosis, no matter the symptoms or personal situation, is more at risk of developing mental health conditions without endometriosis.
Some possible endometriosis-related factors that experts believe could lead to the development of anxiety or depression (among other mental health conditions) are chronic pelvic pain, pain during sex, infertility, time since diagnosis, age, relationship status, supportiveness of intimate partner, and self-perception or self-esteem. This is true of the symptoms the woman is exercising, which may lead to a negative sense of female identity, which may impact a woman's self-esteem and self-perception. Negative self-perception or low self-esteem may then contribute to feelings of anxiety or depression.

However, a study showed that depression was present in 86% of women who experienced severe pain related to endometriosis. 38% of women with little to no pain related to endometriosis experienced depression.

I want to point out I spent many hours fact-checking these facts and statistics, which are acute as of February 4th, 2022. things constantly change, and I hope by the time this book is published and in your hands that there will be a cure; living with Endometriosis, living with any chronic illness doesn't give a life that most people imagine.

One in ten women have Endometriosis which is approximately 176 million women globally, yet only 20% of the general public have heard of Endometriosis. This is so sad and brings many misconceptions to the table, some I will be touching on throughout this book. This book would have thousands of pages worth of information if I were to touch on every single one, so I have picked out ones that I know many suffer get asked.

Endometriosis increases the risk of premature birth by 26% and the need for a Caesarean section by 40%.

Endometriosis is the second most common gynecological condition in the UK. And The financial cost to the world of Endometriosis is similar to that of diabetes. It's estimated to be about US$10,762 per woman per year. Two-thirds of that cost is due to lost work productivity, and the remaining US$3,497 is in direct health care costs.

Endometriosis affects every woman differently, and no one treatment will work for everyone because Endometriosis is still considered taboo even though documents date back over 4,000 years ago with Endometriosis being discovered in a woman. Because Endometriosis is still regarded as taboo, it takes an average of 7.5 years from the onset of symptoms to get a diagnosis.

Endometriosis is not only about painful periods; but they're also are four different stages. And The severity of Endometriosis doesn't necessarily correlate with the amount of pain or other symptoms a woman has.

Many people think Endometriosis is a woman-only disease, yet in sporadic cases, it has been found in males. Other people think it only affects women of reproductive age, but there are significant premenarchal endometriosis cases. Premenarchal Endometriosis is when Endometriosis develops before menstruation begins. A handful of cases of Endometriosis in neonates (newborn infants) have also been reported, which shows no one is too young to have this painful condition.

As of writing this, no one knows the underlying cause of Endometriosis; Because of this, there is no cure for Endometriosis. Many people have the misconception that Both a hysterectomy and

Pregnancy will cure the disease, but that is not true. Just like hormone therapy, it may relieve symptoms but will not cure them.

I have been asked numerous times if I have tried yoga, if I have tried meditating or not focusing on it, and it annoys me almost as much as people telling me that I am too young to be sick or that God will make everything better. I know yoga does work for other women, but I find it annoying to be asked that when I have gone through so many treatments ad tried a lot to manage the pain with nothing working. The recurrence rate after hormonal treatment is 70%.

Something else that annoys me is people asking if they will catch Endometriosis if they hang out with me or saying that sex is only painful because I'm "tight."

The only way to be officially diagnosed is via laparoscopy but even with a specialist
Endometriosis can still come back after your surgery.

Touching on the infertility side of Endometriosis, The percentage of infertility in a woman with Endometriosis can be as high as 30–50%. Having this chronic illness does not guarantee infertility, which doctors need to tell people more about instead of saying they have very little chance of ever having kids.

40% of women with fertility issues have Endometriosis, and Endometriosis doesn't just cause it on the tubes.

Painful periods ARE NOT NORMAL, especially if the pain is severe. A misconception is that Endometriosis is Endometrium (Endometrium is one of the inner lining layers of the uterus and functions to prevent adhesions between the opposed walls of the myometrium)

Most people don't understand that pain can be a daily occurrence, not just around the period, and only 20% of women feel their current pain management is effective. A colossal 33% of women are told the pain, and everything they are experiencing is in their heads.

Endometriosis affects more than just our bodies. 32% of women experience depression due to their Endometriosis, 80% of women miss work because of their condition, and 73% of women have relationships affected because of their Endometriosis

82% of women cannot carry out day-to-day activities because of Endometriosis.

People do not have this because they decided not to breed in their early 20s. Delaying Pregnancy is not a cause of Endometriosis.

Earlier in this book I touched on diet as a way to try and help with Endometriosis but I know a quick google search will bring up so much information that it can be overwhelming.

The Endometriosis diet is one of those diets that everyone globally argues about. Those lucky enough for it to work swear by the diet and say that it is the answer for everything. For those who It doesn't work for, they get annoyed at everyone who pushes the diet, saying it's the answer for everyone or that you didn't stick at it long enough, which is not what you want to hear when in pain That's my experience from what I have seen in our community and through research. However, it might be different in other communities that I am not a part of.
The basics of the Endometriosis diet are to cut out red meat, Trans Fats, caffeine, dairy, alcohol, refined sugars, processed foods, soy, and carbohydrates while eating more Fruits, Vegetables, Whole

Grains, Omega-3 Fats, iron-rich foods, fibrous foods and foods that are rich in essential fatty acids.

A Research study was done a few years back. 75% of participants reported significant reductions in symptom severity after 12 months. They also found that it improved mental health, social function, vitality, physical function, and perceived healthiness after following the diet.

While another study was done, this time with the low FODMAP diet, which has been proven for treating IBS, recent studies suggest that it may help ease endometriosis-related bowel symptoms.

In one study that included 58 women with both Endometriosis and irritable bowel syndrome, 72% of patients saw a significant improvement in bowel symptoms after four weeks on a low FODMAP diet. The success rate for the low FODMAP diet was also significantly higher for women with endometriosis compared to women with just IBS.

There is one problem with diets, though, and it's not the diet itself but those who try and push out the diet by saying it will cure all your issues which is just false. Sometimes an underlying condition causes more problems than just what the Endometriosis is causing. Because there is no cure, The pressure to go onto an Endometriosis diet is misleading; it is set to try and get women to change to this diet in hopes of no longer having endometriosis. This, in turn, affects general public eye information that makes them believe that this diet can cure Endometriosis and that sufferers are over exaggerating.

I Have tried the diet in the past, and while it works for some women, it most definitely doesn't work for me. I found my symptoms worsening because I cut out one of the only things that helped me in pain, sugar.

 I had done this diet while I was very young without even knowing it. As a kid, I couldn't eat gluten or sugar because I would have an allergic reaction, this was for many years, and nothing happened with my Endometriosis even though we didn't know that it was affecting me at the time.

With age, I grew out of my allergy, and I eventually did try the diet outside of my allergies. I find sugar helps with my pain, eating chocolate or lollies helps lessen my pain levels during my period, and the only way I can have a bowel movement is if I have coffee, so it was tough to be on a diet.

Other ladies have had similar experiences as I with the diet, and that is because no blanket option will work for everyone; diets help some people and not others; the same with birth control options and pain killers. Nothing is going to work for every single person, no matter if they suffer chronic illness or not.

It's also why some people go on a diet for weight loss, which either doesn't work, or they gain it all back.

I think changing your lifestyle in some ways definitely has a significant effect on Endometriosis, but it won't cure it, and no one lifestyle change will work for everyone; sadly, it all comes down to trial and error to find what works for you.

For me, caffeine helps with bowel pain, and sugar helps with my cramps, but by exercising a bit more by going on walks or dancing, I find it also helps lessen my bleeding timeframe, which allows how long I am in extreme pain for.

Having spent my teen years suffering from this harsh and painful condition, I had to go through my whole dating life in physical and mental pain. I will admit I did start dating a lot earlier in my life than most, which looking back on, I wish I hadn't done, but in doing so, I learned what I wanted in a relationship early on and learned a lot of stuff in the process.

Throughout my early dating life, I didn't know I had endometriosis. All I knew was that I was in horrible pain. Most of the people I dated didn't last past the four-month mark, and none ever made it past seven months. This was the case even after we found out I had suspected endometriosis.

Guys and girls alike never really understood it, even when I was full-on crying and vomiting from the pain. Things were said like
"sex isn't painful, don't be a baby,"
"come on, let's go out and do something," "Hunny, it's just cramping; I get them too. They aren't that bad; just Toughen up."

One guy I was dating always had me at the gym, which when I wasn't on my period or ovulating was okay because I didn't have to do any strenuous workouts.
I would generally walk on the treadmill, lift weights or do leg presses and just stop and take a break when I was getting sore.

When we first started dating, I warned him from the get-go that I had previously experienced problems with moving and getting out of bed from the pain. Luckily the three months we were together, I didn't have that problem, just loads of bloating no matter how much I worked out or did and didn't eat, which led to him body-shaming me throughout the whole time and calling me a liar for saying I had experienced things in the past that never happened when we were together.

In the early making of this book, I got into another relationship after being single for over a year. I warned him like I always did before I got in a relationship with anyone because It is better for them to know and be prepared for the worst-case scenario and it not happen than not tell them, and it happens, and they go, what the fuck and leave.

The guy who was body-shaming me gave me some very unwanted advice when he randomly messaged me out of the blue, and I brought up the fact that I was going on a date. These almost exact words were, "don't say you can't work or walk around at times" he then followed up by saying, "have you gotten a real job yet?" now, let's address this really quick, I was fourteen and fifteen when he and I were dating, I had two jobs in the past one like a calf rearer, and one was a volunteering job in primary and middle school restocking shelves at an eco-friendly store and a few babysitting jobs here and there, so straight away working at that age was very unlikely for anyone. I know some people do, but the mass majority don't. Most are focused on school so that they are set to work in the future, and writing a book and running a youtube channel is most definitely real work, especially when you get paid to do it; by the time we were dating, I had self-published one book and sold a few copies. It later went off the market, and I was getting paid from my youtube at the time.

I never said I couldn't work in a 'regular job' as he put it, just that it would be challenging and I would be pushing through a lot of pain, And just because he or any other guy doesn't see the pain, I am in, or the bad days I go through.

The days I couldn't walk (the person I dated before he saw me not getting out of bed) doesn't mean it doesn't happen or hasn't happened in the past.

I have always found it hard to tell guys and girls because so many people don't know about it and assume what they see is it, which any suffer knows is bullshit. This condition is on the inside, making it invisible the only symptoms you see are the ones you are around to see, like vomiting from pain; even then, people will tell you to suck it up and get on with life. Which yes, we don't need to allow it to control our lives, but it's easier said than done, especially since the pain can change throughout the day, making it near impossible to make plans, and when we do, we may need to cancel them.

My first date with my now ex-boyfriend at the time of writing this was at a restaurant for breakfast; I was hungry that day which isn't normal for me in the mornings, so I ordered my favourite thing they make. But I was barely able to eat much of it at the time (I did finish it later that day) because the minute I started eating, I felt sick to my stomach and was on the verge of throwing up. I remember texting my mum almost in tears because he kept giving me strange looks. After all, I kept gagging on my food. Thankfully that relationship didn't end because of my endometriosis, but we definitely had our ups and downs with it.

I was lucky enough, however, to get into some good relationships, one of which was a long-distance relationship with a South African boy who I will forever hold dear to my heart and the other with my current partner, who, from day one, has supported everything.

Friendships can also be affected, while not because of the lack of sex or sexual affection.

I don't even remember how many times I had made plans and was unable to make it, so I had to cancel the plan's with my friends because those days, the pain was so bad that I was stuck in a hot bath or bed all day.

It is no secret I have anger issues. Pain makes my anger shoot through the roof, so many augments happened, or they physically didn't understand. I ended the friendship because they thought I was faking being in pain for attention; some even went as far as to copycat to try and get attention for themselves.

Everything needs communication, but when people don't understand or don't want to understand that, they will sometimes say it's all excuses to be challenging.

Because of all of this, I stopped making friends and just became a lone wolf in a sense; because it is just too hard to spend a year or two on a friendship and have to cancel plans one time after pushing myself through all the other hang out sessions and had to deal with the consequent that night and the next day. I know they were not real friends, but you never know until it happens, so I just gave up.

At one stage, I did date a guy who came out of nowhere which is the father of my child, but in the end, it didn't work out because of my mental health caused by childhood trauma and my endometriosis. I tried my hardest to get everything in control, but other issues within the relationship caused it not to work out.

Dating with endometriosis shouldn't be as challenging as it is, but it is making friends with endometriosis shouldn't be hard. Still, it is endometriosis that doesn't just affect your body and mind. It affects your workability, your ability to maintain friendships and relationships it impacts the range of dating possibilities; it shouldn't define us this much, but it does for a lot of us, which isn't helpful at all when all you want is love that something you can't even help has taken that away from you.

The right guy or girl is there for everyone, but it's finding them. The dating world is so hard that it's just full of regrets and people not understanding, which puts the sufferer at a standstill of whether it's worth pursuing to find the right person who will hold onto them and help them through their pain days.

My daughter's father, I thought, was like that, and he was accommodating. We just didn't work. He wasn't the man for me at the time. But he showed me they were good guys out there who would accept me for my endometriosis and flaws. I am now working on myself a lot more to try for my next relationship if it ever comes to be the best person I can be so that when I am in large amounts of pain, my small anger bursts doesn't define the whole relationship I'm not saying dead in that relationship either. Still, I know my anger and how I react to the pain doesn't help in relationships in general.

As with everything in life, there are risks associated. Risk factors of endometriosis depend on how severe the endometriosis is.

some risks that could signal you may be at risk for having endometriosis:
Family history of endometriosis,
getting your period early in life,
Short menstrual cycles (< 27 d),
Long duration of menstrual flow (>7 d),
Heavy bleeding during period,
Defects in the uterus or fallopian tube.

some risks that can come from having endometriosis:
infertility,
Debilitating pelvic pain,
Adhesions,
ovarian cysts,
loss of work,
higher risk of clear cell ovarian cancer and endometrioid ovarian cancer,
Impaired uterine artery flow.

There are so many risks associated with this illness, but those are just some of them. The day-to-day struggles depend on the woman and the time of the month. I am in pain daily for someone like me, and it affects how long I can sit upright, my walking at times, my eating habits, and more.

Those with sexual partners who experience pain during intercourse affect their sex lives and pleasure.
For someone on their period, it can affect going out due to heavy bleeding and pain. Those with jobs can affect their work-life

because of flare-ups, so you have to have an understanding boss for when you need to head home.

There are countless ways it affects people, and if I was to list all of them, this book is hundreds of pages long, but because it depends on the woman, some will have all of these and more. In contrast, others may not have any struggles other than pain due to several factors from personal pain level, stage, and more.

I get asked specific questions a lot, and while working on this book, I did several polls and questionnaires to find out what people wanted to know to make the best of this book and some questions I have covered throughout the book. Still, I got asked by the general public and friends, so I decided to address them here.

Q. does it affect you daily.
A. as I have said before, endometriosis affects everyone differently, and I can only speak for myself. But yes, for me, endometriosis affects me daily.

Q. what tests do you go through to find out.
A. the only for sure way to know you have endometriosis is by laparoscopy. Even then, they can miss it if it is hidden, and that is why some woman still push after surgery shows nothing because they know something else is wrong. Typically you will be sent for ultrasounds to try and see if anything is visible; they will rarely see anything on an ultrasound.

Q. how to relieve symptoms.
A. every person is different in this aspect, but things like pain medications, heat, cold, and weighted blankets can help. To work out what benefits you will be found with trial and error. Like I found when I am feeling sick because of endometriosis, anti-nausea pills work wonders.

Q. What is endometriosis.
A. endometriosis is a condition in which the lining of the uterus doesn't shead like it is meant to

Q. Does Endometriosis just affect the pelvic region
A.Now the most common place for Endometriosis is the pelvic region, but this horrible condition spreads like fire all around the body and has even been found in the lungs and brain.

Q. can you prevent Endometriosis
A.Because there is not much known about Endometriosis and no one knows why Endometriosis occurs, there is no way to prevent yourself from getting Endometriosis, there are treatments for the management of symptoms and to try and slow the growth and spread, but they don't work for everyone.

Q. Which organ is most commonly Affected by Endometriosis
A.Endometriosis most commonly involves your ovaries, fallopian tubes and the tissue lining your pelvis.

Q.What causes endometriosis
A.The exact cause of endometriosis is unknown, but several theories offer possible explanations. When a woman has her period, some of the blood and tissue from her uterus travels out through the fallopian tubes and into the pelvis and very rarely other areas of the body. This is called retrograde menstruation. Nearly all women have some degree of retrograde menstruation, so abnormalities of the endometrial tissue in the uterus, a receptive environment in the pelvis, and alterations in the local immune system likely contribute to the development of endometriosis. Other theories exist to explain endometriosis lesions in rare locations outside of the pelvis, and researchers are actively exploring other causes.

Q.Do I need to have a hysterectomy?
A.No, a hysterectomy is not necessary. However, if a woman with endometriosis is not interested in becoming pregnant, she and her doctor may decide to remove the uterus and possibly the ovaries if other treatments are ineffective.

Q.Is endometriosis a form of cancer?
A.No, endometriosis is not a type of cancer. Some research suggests that women with endometriosis may be at a slightly higher risk of developing certain cancers.

Q.Can endometriosis be inherited?
A.The condition often affects members of the same nuclear family, such as sisters, mothers, and grandmothers. People with cousins who have the condition are also at an increased risk. Endometriosis can be inherited via the maternal or paternal family line, but the link is still being studied.

Q. Can you have kids with endometriosis?
Yea, while some people may struggle to get pregnant and have an increased risk of not being able to get pregnant. many women get pregnant with Endometriosis and go full term and have healthy, happy babies

At the beginning of writing this book, I created a survey on survey monkey; A website where you can produce free surveys and share the link online to get a range of responses that are all in one place for easy viewing. I asked other sufferers ten questions in total, all of which they could skip if they didn't feel comfortable answering something.

The questions were.

1- Have you been officially diagnosed with Endometriosis?

2- How old were you when diagnosed?
3- How many surgeries have you had?
4- What do you wish people knew about Endometriosis?
5- What was your first symptom, and at what age?
6- How do you manage the pain?
7- Did/does the Endometriosis diet help you?
8- How old are you now?
9- Any other comments you want to be included, please add what you want your name to be displayed as in the book?
10- Are you okay with your answers being written up and published in my book?

Some people didn't want their names included, so they will be known as -Anon {age} and everyone who didn't want their answers included has been skipped in respect to them. I had over thirty-three submissions and have only included twenty-six of the submissions.

Yes, I have been officially diagnosed. I was thirty-eight when I was finally diagnosed, which was twenty-five years after the onset of my symptoms which all started when I was thirteen years old. I have had two surgeries for my Endometriosis. I really want people to know how hard it can be to be taken seriously medically. I manage my pain with Drugs, mindfulness, friends, so I don't really manage it at all. I haven't tried the endo diet. I sought out a hysterectomy when I was thirty-four due to clots, flooding, pain (!!!!) and more and was told that the Dr would not do it because I might meet a man and he might want children. This despite my loss of twins, my history of miscarriage, and me telling her I had a living daughter and had completed my family. I was so shocked. At thirty-eight, I was diagnosed with Endometriosis, Adenomyosis and hallmarked for Endometrial cancer. A hysterectomy was rushed. - Anon 38

I was officially diagnosed at 18 after I started having really painful periods at seventeen, so I thankfully only had to wait a year for my diagnosis. I have had four surgeries in total, and I want people to know how painful and chronic it is all the time. I use pain medication and hot water bottles to manage my pain I am also cautious about what I eat, which helps with my symptoms - Tracey 43

My first symptom was terrible back pain when I was nineteen, and I was officially diagnosed when I was thirty-three. I have only ever had my diagnostic surgery. I wish people knew that you have pain between periods. I used to have pain every time I ate before I started using the endo diet. I use an anti-inflammatory diet also known as the Endometriosis diet, exercise, Ibuprofen, Panadol and Tramadol to manage my pain and symptoms - Anon 34

When I was around sixteen, I started to have immense bowel pain when I was going toilet, I have now had three surgery's, and I was diagnosed at twenty-two. I wish people knew that it isn't just bad period pain and that there is no cure. Having a baby may help, but the symptoms return, and by the time we go to the doctors, we have had years and years of pain, and we are not attention seekers or druggies. We just want relief. I manage my pain with over the counter medication and the Endometriosis diet - Anna P 34

I have tried everything at some point to manage my pain, Amitriptyline, opioids, medically induced menopause. I even tried the endo diet, and it didn't help me. My first symptom presented at twelve years old with severe bleeds and pain. I was finally diagnosed at eighteen and have had twenty-five surgeries. I wish people knew how pervasive and exhausting it is also limit the number of "exploratory and laser" laparoscopic procedures. The price you pay for excess surgery in the form of adhesions isn't worth the temporary respite -Anon 44

My first symptom was Irregular, painful periods that made me bedridden since they commenced at thirteen. I was diagnosed at twenty-seven, and I manage the pain with Ibuprofen, heat packs, Showers and sleep. I wish people knew that although you can't see it, It's real, and the pain is real. There are good days and bad days and days where you can not do anything. - Anon 30

At twenty-seven, I started having pain and bleeding. I manage my pain with Advil. I was diagnosed at twenty-seven and have had two surgeries so far. I wish people knew to have painful and debilitating it is. - Anon 44

I manage my pain with a pain management clinic, dieting (FODMAP has helped identify my trigger foods for inflammation), exercise and alternative medicines. My symptoms started at eleven, and I was diagnosed at fifteen. I have now had eight surgeries. I wish people knew that chronic pain is a non-visible disability. - Devon Clark 28

I was diagnosed at twenty-one, and I have had five surgeries. my first symptom started at thirteen, which was extremely heavy and painful periods. I wish people knew how debilitating the pain can be. I use heat packs and painkillers to try and manage my pain, but most of the time, that doesn't work.- Ange Solway 41

I use the Endometriosis diet, and I know if I stick to it, it works, but as soon as I have something I shouldn't, I notice very quickly. Sugar is probably the worst for me. I also use Tramadol, lyrical and have just started using CBD to manage my pain which began at twelve years old. I remember my first period being very painful and the doctor telling me it was all in my head, but I finally got answers at thirty-three. I wish people knew that excruciating pain is not normal and that it can be hereditary. My mother has it and probably had the answers to my pain all along. now I fear my daughter will suffer the same pain I have all these years. -Nerissa 36

I was diagnosed at twenty-four. A week prior, my uterus becoming engorged. I was diagnosed when I had my emergency hysterectomy. I wish people knew that Endometriosis is more than just cramps, and doctors need to realize the pain is real. I just power through the pain.- Sara H. 37

I mange my pain with Codiene, paracetamol, trasnanamic acid and oramorph. I have tried diets and haven't found any that help. My first symptom was extreme vaginal bleeding from age twelve. People need to know just how painful it is and just how awful it is when you are bleeding more than a patient being rushed into hospital; to still hear it's just a period. I was diagnosed at twenty-five.- Front-line warrior 26

I was diagnosed at thirty-two and have had seven surgeries for this god awful condition. My first symptoms were when I was twenty years old, and I was getting sore ribs, bad backaches and became extremely tired. I use Ice packs, hot showers, medical marijuana, oxycodone, and sleep to manage the pain. I have noticed the Endometriosis diet helps I am sixteen weeks into it as of answering this questionnaire, and I have fewer bloat and IBS (Irritable bowel syndrome) symptoms. the pain from Endometriosis is how I imagine dying feels. - Anon 39

People need to know that this is real; it is painful all the time. It ruins lives, jobs and relationships. I was twenty-four when I was diagnosed, and I started having agonizing pain around the age of twenty-three/ twenty-four. I am currently using nothing to manage my pain because the doctors won't prescribe me anything. we need the proper research. I am from the UK, and none of my local hospitals knows much about Endometriosis. it's not in my head; I

am not crazy; I am human; I am in pain, listen to me, believe me. -
Anon 26

I have had two surgeries for this condition and was diagnosed at
twenty-one. My first symptom was pain at fourteen. People need to
know it is extremely painful. I use the Endometriosis diet and
cannabis to manage my pain. -Kristen McRobie (founder of
Endometriosis and me) 30

People need to know That it's not just 'bad period pains' and how
many other aspects of your health is affected. I had always had
irregular and very painful periods, but from thirty-five onwards, the
pain was ridiculous for weeks at a time, and I was finally diagnosed
at thirty-eight. I also have IBS (Irritable bowel syndrome), and I use
a hot water bottle and lots of pain killers to try and help the pain. -
Beth Arrandale 40

I just want people to know that for the women who have this, we
need good support systems who believe our pain and are willing to
stick by us even when we are having a flare-up for the second week
in a row and can't do what we normally do. This disease drains you
of energy, self-confidence, and dreams. This condition hurts, and
when I can't get out of bed from the pain, it is real. I'm not just lazy;
I was diagnosed at eighteen and have had five surgeries.-Katelin
Frybarger 24

I was 13 years when I started my third period. My belly was bloated,
and I was extremely sick and had to go to schools that day: I ended
up puking at school and got sent home and was bed rested for the
rest of the day, including the following day. I was finally diagnosed
at twenty-three. I try and tough out the pain, but that doesn't
always work. people need to know that it is slow torture; this is
serious, and it is not something to pass up.-Nibbler 24

The endo diet has helped me somewhat, and I also use CBD and THC to manage my pain. I was thirteen years old; I had heavy bleeding and pain since I've started menstruating. I was first diagnosed at twenty-four and have currently had nine surgeries. just because we look okay on the outside doesn't mean we aren't in pain.-Tammy T 41

At age eighteen, I started with a hemorrhaging ovarian cyst; my doctor saw signs of endo. Two years later, with irregular period, I am in stage one. Lesions are on the lining of my uterus. This is the second hormonal treatment I'm on, and just hoping for the best. I manage my pain using hormonal treatments and lots of strong painkillers; sometimes, the pain is so strong and unbearable there's no choice but to go to the ER. And I'm from the Caribbean as well. All the way from Trinidad. I found the Endometriosis diet doesn't really help me because there are lots of fruits and veggies I'm not allowed to eat because it easily triggers everything. I was diagnosed at eighteen, and people need to know how painful it is. The effect Endometriosis causes on your body. How it impacts your life; physically, emotionally and mentally. - Sid_the_trini_living_with_endo. 21

The Endometriosis diet didn't help me. I don't really manage my pain; I take painkillers just to make daily life bearable I have had fourteen surgeries, and I was diagnosed at nineteen. I started having heavy bleeding and pain at fourteen. people need to understand how bad it actually is, and it is not just exaggerating period pains-Caroline 42

Since doing the Endometriosis diet, I have noticed my bloating is a lot less. To manage pain, I use water bottles, pain killers and taking time off school. I was twelve when my symptoms started, and I was officially diagnosed at thirty-two. The larger-scale effects associated with the disease. Fatigue. hormone imbalance issues like acne, foggy brain, conditions more than likely to develop as a result of taking strong drugs like Zoladex, birth control pills, NSAIDs -Anon 40

Women are strong and resilient, and often health professionals don't take "women's issues" seriously and advise stuff like iron tablets and contraception. Women should stand strong; if YOU want a referral, YOU should get it. ALL options of treatment should be offered, from medications to surgeries, depending on what YOU want. The public health sector needs improved funding for women's health to enable everyone to have access to good quality care as not everyone can afford an insurance policy. I've had heavy, painful periods my whole menstrual life (since I was twelve), so I couldn't really say what my first symptom was, but it was only ever mentioned when I had a couple of years of infertility then I had my diagnosis and surgery after seeing a new fertility specialist as unable to conceive for ten years. I was thirty-eight when it was discovered. People need to know that it doesn't just affect your period; it is present throughout the whole month. Also, most women "forget" how bad their pain is because it becomes our norm, and we just carry on with this as much as possible. also, medical professionals may suspect a woman has it for many years and not be in too much of a bother actually to investigate it more. -Leah B 39

I was fifteen when I thought the heavy periods with pains might not be normal. At the moment, I am at the point that I just deal with the pain because pain killers don't seem to help. I just wish more doctors would properly listen to you and not make you feel like you are attention-seeking. doctors and other people need to know how debilitating it actually is and that it's not "in your head" -Jade M 26

People need to know how much different you feel day to day; You may feel like a million bucks today, and that all can change with one wrong move. I have now have had six surgeries, and I was diagnosed at seventeen.-Melissa Corbeil 27

Endometriosis is a disease that can stop women from living normal everyday lives. Interfere with every aspect of life. I was diagnosed at sixteen. My first memory of having this condition was at around thirteen to fourteen years old, and all I remember is kneeling over in pain a lot. I have had six surgeries. I try to manage it; I have a marina IUD and take painkillers when needed. It never seems to get on top of the pain totally, though, and I can't always take morphine for daily flare-ups. I wouldn't wish this disease on my worst enemy. I have lived with Endometriosis for twenty odd years now, and I still can't "manage" my pain. Well, it becomes a matter of putting one foot in front of the other most days, especially since I am a solo mum to a young daughter, so I just have to keep going -Anon 36

Thank you to all the ladies who answered. You are all strong, and hopefully, soon, we will have the funding, research and cure that we need. It is not right that we live the way we do, especially with all the judgement we get.

Here are the references that I used to make this book

https://www.bbc.com/news/health-33115478#targetText=A%20study%2C%20on%20nearly%2015%2C000,%25%20and%2010%25%20of%20women.
http://nezhat.org/endometriosis-of-young-girls-and-teenagers/
http://endometriosis.org/news/research/long-term-effect-on-physical-mental-and-social-wellbeing-due-to-endometriosis/
https://www.theguardian.com/society/2015/sep/28/endometriosis-20-things-every-woman-and-every-doctor-should-know#targetText=The%20financial%20cost%20to%20the,is%20in%20direct%20healthcare%20costs.
http://nezhat.org/endometriosis-treatment/history-of-endometriosis/
http://nezhat.org/endometriosis-of-young-girls-and-teenagers/
http://www.fertilityandpregnancyedinburgh.com/blog/how-to-manage-your-endometriosis-better-with-these-12-tips
http://www.endostats.com/advocacy/endostats-was-created-to-simplify-endometriosis-information

http://www.idph.state.il.us/about/womenshealth/factsheets/endo.
htm#targetText=In%20what%20places%2C%20outside%20of,behin
d%20the%20uterus